BREASTFEEDING
Keep It Simple

Second Edition

Amy Spangler, MN, RN, IBCLC

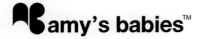

Production

Cover Design: thehappycorp global, thehappycorp.com, New York, New York, USA

Cover Photography: Doctor Jaeger, doctorjaeger.com, New York, New York, USA

Editing and Interior Design: Carol Adams Rivera, MA, Health Communication Connection, healthcommunication.info, Vienna, Virginia, USA

Illustrations: Rick Powell, studiopowell.com, Montpelier, Vermont, USA

Printing: Specialty Lithographing Co., Cincinnati, Ohio, USA

Second Edition

12 11 10 09 08 07 06   1 2 3 4 5

ISBN 1-933634-02-2

For families everywhere

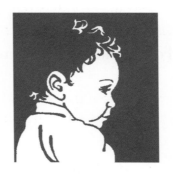

Learning to breastfeed
is like learning to ride a bicycle—
it may seem hard at first, but once you learn,
it is simple!

There are a few things you need
to know before you begin…

Be patient!
Some babies know how to breastfeed right away,
but most need to learn.

Be persistent!
It may take several days or several weeks before
you and your baby know just what to do.

Be proud!
You are giving your baby a gift that lasts forever.

What is in this book?

Deciding to Breastfeed

Getting Ready to Breastfeed

Beginning to Breastfeed

Taking Care of Your Baby

Breastfeeding Special Babies

Taking Care of Yourself

Returning to Work or School

Getting Help

Author's Notes
Throughout this book the baby is referred to as *he*
or *him.*

Elephants never forget and neither should you! A picture
of an elephant is used throughout this book to point out
important information you need to remember to keep
your baby healthy and safe.

Deciding to Breastfeed

Why should I breastfeed?

Breastfeeding is the safest and simplest way to feed your baby. It makes life easier for the whole family!

Breastfed babies are healthier! Breastfed babies have...

- fewer ear infections.
- less gas, constipation, and diarrhea.
- less risk of pneumonia.
- less risk of allergy and asthma.
- less risk of sudden infant death syndrome (SIDS).
- less risk of obesity in childhood.
- less risk of diabetes.

Breastfed babies are happier! Breastfed babies...

- get to know you right away.
- feel safe in your arms.

Breastfed babies are smarter! Babies who breastfeed...

- have better brain development.
- do better on IQ tests.

Mothers who breastfeed are healthier! Mothers who breastfeed have...

- less bleeding after childbirth and lose weight sooner.
- less risk of breast, ovarian, and uterine cancer.
- strong bones.

Breastfeeding saves time and money! Parents who breastfeed...

- save more than $1,000 (US) the first year alone by not having to buy bottles, nipples, and formula.
- miss fewer days of work and lose less income.

Breastmilk is the perfect food for your baby! Breastmilk...

- contains more than 200 nutrients.
- is always ready.
- is clean and safe.
- is never too hot or too cold.
- makes vaccines work better.

Breastfeeding makes your life simpler and easier!

What should I do if my family and friends tell me not to breastfeed?

Learn all that you can about breastfeeding before your baby is born. Share this knowledge with family and friends. Let them know that breastfeeding is BEST for you and your baby. Be sure to tell grandma how much you need her help as you learn to be a mother to her grandchild.

How can I breastfeed in front of others without feeling uneasy?

Some mothers are uncomfortable breastfeeding in front of others. Some are not. If you live in a place where breasts are seen mostly as sex objects, you may be shy about breastfeeding in public. It may help to remember that breastfeeding is what breasts were meant to do. With a little practice, you can learn to breastfeed without your breasts showing. Let your partner know that you need his support. Be confident! You are giving your baby the very best.

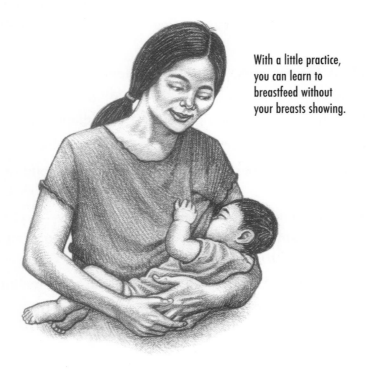

With a little practice, you can learn to breastfeed without your breasts showing.

Will my partner feel left out?

Breastfeeding benefits everyone who is a part of your baby's life. Breastfed babies have fewer doctor visits and hospital stays, making parenting easier. Nighttime feedings are simple when there is no formula to mix, measure, or warm. Breastfed babies are portable—good news for families on the go!

Breastfeeding does take time and energy, especially in the early weeks. It is easy for partners—especially fathers—to get discouraged. Fortunately the early weeks are short-lived. Let your partner know how much you need his support as you learn to care for your baby.

Hints for partners, especially fathers
- Learn all you can about breastfeeding.
- Help with positioning, burping, and diapering.
- Feed your partner while she feeds your baby.
- Let your partner know that you are very proud of her.
- Spend time alone each day with your baby—go for a walk, splash in the tub, sing, dance, read, or simply watch TV together.
- If you feel jealous or angry, talk about your feelings.
- Spend time alone each week with your partner!

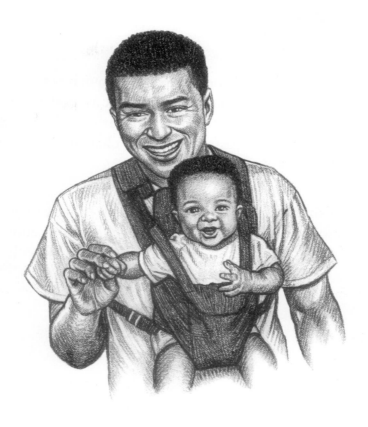

Spending time together is the best way to get to know your baby.

Are my breasts too small for me to breastfeed?

Breasts come in all shapes and sizes. Women with small breasts produce just as much milk as women with large breasts. Most babies will learn to breastfeed on their mother's breasts if given the chance. All it takes is practice!

Nipple size and shape can make breastfeeding easier or harder for some babies. If you have questions about the size or shape of your breasts or nipples, talk with your health care provider.

Will breastfeeding change the size and shape of my breasts?

You may find that your breasts get smaller after your baby is born and the weight that you gained during pregnancy is lost. This can happen no matter how you choose to feed your baby.

Does breastfeeding hurt?

Breastfeeding should not hurt if your baby is positioned well. You may feel pulling or tugging at the start of a feeding when your baby latches on to your breast. Some mothers say this pulling or tugging is painful, but it should last only a few seconds. If it lasts more than a few seconds, break the suction by sliding your finger into your baby's mouth. Take your baby off the breast, and try again.

How much time does breastfeeding take?

In the beginning, babies eat often, but this gives you and your baby a chance to spend time together and get to know one another!

Getting Ready to Breastfeed

How does the breast make milk?

There are special cells inside the breast that make milk. Small tubes, called *milk ducts*, carry the milk from the milk-producing cells to openings in the nipple.

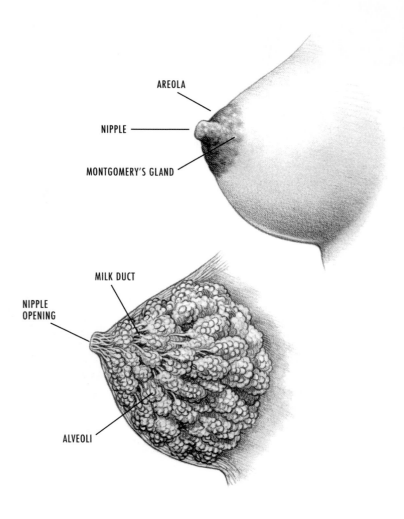

AREOLA

NIPPLE

MONTGOMERY'S GLAND

MILK DUCT

NIPPLE OPENING

ALVEOLI

When your baby breastfeeds, a message is sent to your brain: "I'm hungry!" Your brain hears the message and signals your breasts to release milk. This release of milk from the breasts is called the *let-down reflex*. You may feel tingling or burning in your breasts when your milk lets down. Or you may see milk dripping from your nipples. Don't worry if you feel or see nothing. Every mother is different.

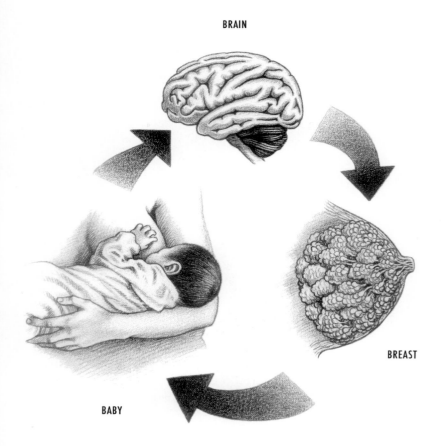

BRAIN

BREAST

BABY

Your brain also signals your breasts to make more milk to replace the milk your baby takes.

 The more milk your baby removes from your breasts, the more milk you will make.

What does human milk look like?

Colostrum is the first milk your breasts will make. It can be thick and yellow or clear and runny. Colostrum is made during the last months of pregnancy and the first days after birth. New babies need small amounts of food often. So mothers produce small amounts of colostrum each day. Colostrum helps your baby poop, protects your baby from illness, and satisfies your baby's hunger and thirst. Colostrum is your baby's first immunization.

Colostrum is the only food your baby needs.

During the first 2 weeks after birth, your milk will gradually change from colostrum to mature milk. Mature milk has two parts, foremilk and hindmilk. Foremilk is thin and runny. Hindmilk is thick and creamy. Your baby gets foremilk at the start of a feeding and hindmilk at the end of a feeding. Foremilk and hindmilk have all the vitamins, minerals, and nutrients your baby needs to grow.

How do I care for my breasts?

Breasts and nipples require little or no care. *Montgomery's glands*, small pimple-like bumps in the darker part of the breast around the nipple, produce an oily substance that keeps the nipples clean and moist.

Once you are breastfeeding, follow these simple suggestions....

- Wash your breasts once a day when you bathe or shower.

- Use only clear water and mild soap. Do not use lotions, creams, or oils.

- You do not need to wear a bra while breastfeeding, but if you want to wear a bra for comfort or support, you may find a nursing bra handy. Choose a cotton bra that is easy to adjust and fits comfortably.

- If you wear breast pads to protect your clothes, remember to change them often. Choose pads made from soft layers of cotton, silk, or wool cloth. Do not use pads with plastic liners that trap wetness. Some pads are made to be used only once; others can be washed and used again.

- If your skin gets dry, you can use a small amount of modified lanolin. A little bit goes a long way.

- If your nipples are tender, put a few drops of breast-milk on the nipples and areolas after each breast-feeding.

- If you have painful, cracked, or bleeding nipples, call your health care provider for help!

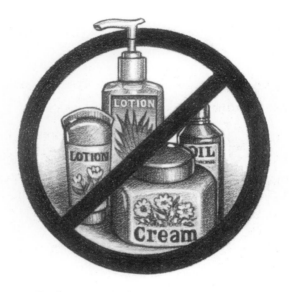

Avoid putting cream, lotion, or oil on your breasts.

Beginning to Breastfeed

How do I get started?

Breastfeed right after your baby is born. Early, frequent feedings will help you and your baby get off to a good start.

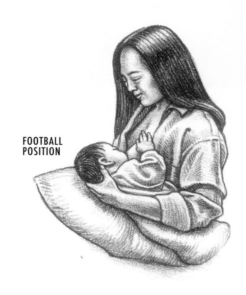

FOOTBALL
POSITION

SIDELYING
POSITION

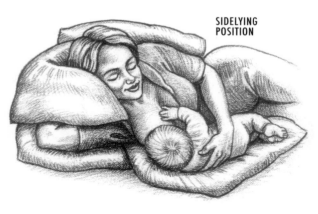

Choose a comfortable position. Place your baby at the level of your breast using pillows for support. Turn your baby on his side or tuck him under your arm so that his head, shoulders, knees, and chest face your breast. Think about how you face the table to eat your meals and position your baby in the same way.

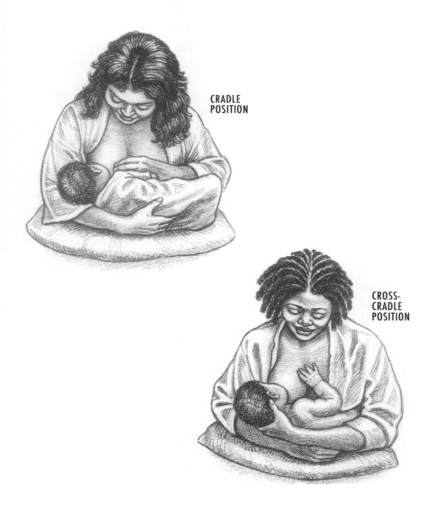

CRADLE
POSITION

CROSS-
CRADLE
POSITION

Express (squeeze out) a few drops of colostrum.
Place your thumb and fingers opposite one another
on the *areola,* the darker part of the breast around the
nipple. Press in against your chest. Then compress
(gently squeeze) the breast, not the nipple, between
your thumb and fingers.

Support your breast. If you need to support your
breast with your hand, make sure you place your
thumb and fingers back away from the nipple.

Support your baby. Place your hand around your
baby's neck for support. Do not place your hand on
the back of your baby's head.

Tickle your baby's nose with your nipple. When his
mouth opens wide, like he is yawning, place him gently
on your breast, starting with his chin and lower lip.
Make sure he has a good, deep latch and a mouth full
of breast!

Hold your baby close and snug. If you hold your
baby close, he will be able to latch on well and compress your breast between the roof of his mouth above
and his tongue below.

Check your baby's nose, cheeks, chin, and lips. Your
baby's chin should press firmly into your breast. His

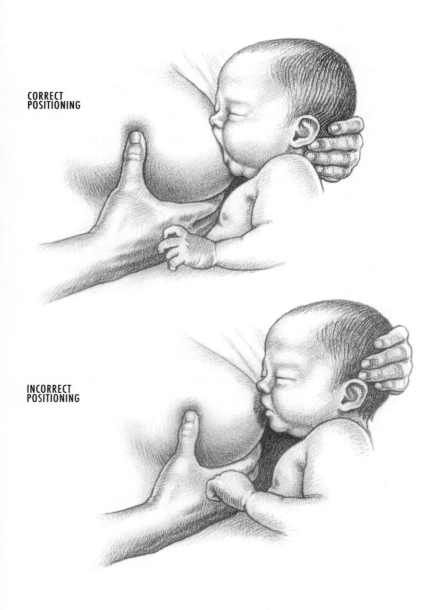

CORRECT
POSITIONING

INCORRECT
POSITIONING

nose and cheeks may lightly touch the breast. His mouth should be opened wide like he is yawning, and his lips should curl out like the lips of a fish!

Watch your baby, not the clock! Breastfeed as long as your baby wishes on the first breast before you offer the second breast (about 10–20 minutes). When your baby stops suckling and swallowing or falls asleep, wake him, burp him, and offer the second breast.

Break the suction before you take your baby off the breast. You can break the suction by gently sliding your finger between your baby's gums and into his mouth.

Offer both breasts at every feeding, but don't worry if your baby seems content with one breast.

Begin each feeding on the breast offered last.

Feed your baby often. Because your baby's stomach is about the same size as his fist, small, frequent feedings are best.

Wait until you and your baby have learned to breastfeed before you offer a bottle or pacifier. Bottle nipples and pacifiers can confuse your baby.

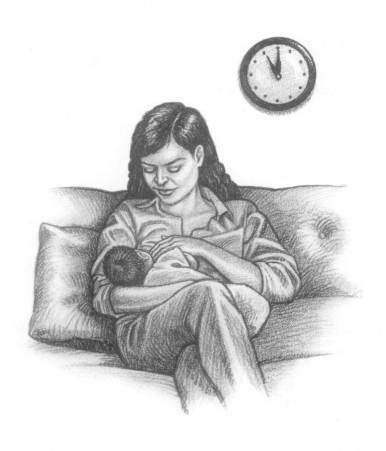

Watch your baby, not the clock!

Relax and enjoy this time with your baby!

 Your breastmilk has all the nutrients your baby needs. If you give your baby water, formula, or other foods, you will make less milk.

How often should I breastfeed?

Breastfeed whenever your baby shows signs of hunger or thirst. These signs include

- squirming
- sucking on hands or fingers
- smacking lips
- coughing
- yawning

Some babies breastfeed every 1–3 hours day and night; others breastfeed every hour for three to five feedings then sleep for 3–4 hours in between. Every baby is different.

Your baby needs to breastfeed at least 8 times in each 24 hours. Many babies breastfeed 10–12 times a day.

Sometimes a sleepy baby will not ask to eat often enough, and you will need to wake him to breastfeed. During the first 4–6 weeks, if your baby does not wake to eat at least eight times in each 24 hours, watch for early signs of hunger or light sleep. Offer the breast at these times. The more milk your baby takes, the more milk you will make.

Hints for waking a sleepy baby

- Place him in your lap in a sitting position and talk to him.
- Massage his feet and back.
- Remove his diaper.
- Wipe his bottom with a cool washcloth.

How long does a feeding last?

Your baby will let you know when he is done!

Some babies breastfeed 10–15 minutes on each breast, some breastfeed 15–30 minutes on each breast, and others breastfeed 15–30 minutes on one breast only.

When your baby stops feeding, burp him and offer the second breast. If he breastfeeds poorly on the first breast, put him back on the first breast before you offer the second breast, so that you can be sure your baby gets the fat and calories he needs to grow. Don't worry if he breastfeeds on only one breast. Each breast can provide a full meal!

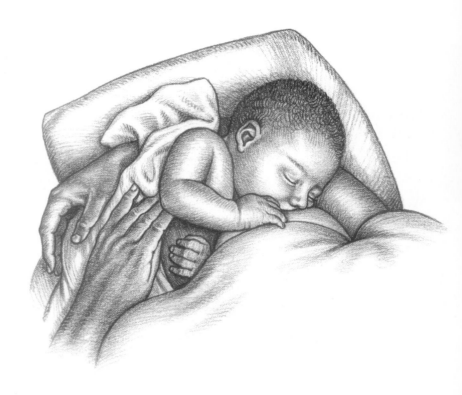

Your baby will let you know when he is done.

Taking Care
of Your Baby

How can I tell if my baby is getting enough to eat?

Many mothers worry about whether their baby is getting enough to eat. Your baby's stomach is the size of his fist, so making enough milk to fill his stomach is easy! Just remember, nothing comes out the bottom unless something goes in the top! You can be sure your baby is getting enough to eat if your baby is

- active and alert.
- happy and satisfied after breastfeeding.
- breastfeeding at least eight times in each 24 hours.
- suckling and swallowing while breastfeeding.
- losing less than 7 percent of his birth weight.
- gaining 4–8 ounces each week after the first week.
- having four or more poops and six or more wet diapers a day by day 5.
- having yellow poop by day 5.
- having clear or pale yellow urine.

If you see *all* these signs, you can be sure your baby is getting enough to eat.

If you are unsure, keep breastfeeding, and call your baby's health care provider or your WIC clinic (see "What is WIC," p. 95).

What should my baby's stool look like?

The good news is that breastfed babies' poop doesn't smell bad.

The bad news is that there is lots of it!

Breastfed babies' stool looks like a mixture of water, yellow mustard, cottage cheese, and sesame seeds. Sometimes a yellow stain the size of your baby's fist is all that you see.

Most babies have four or more stools a day for many weeks. As your baby grows, the size and number of stools will change. Older babies often have fewer but larger stools.

Can I sleep with my baby?

When mothers and babies sleep near one another, nighttime feedings are easier, mothers get more sleep, and babies have less risk of sudden infant death syndrome (SIDS). Babies often sleep in more than one place, including car seats, cribs, cots, bassinets, co-sleepers (baby beds that attach to the side of adult beds), and adult beds. While some sleep areas are safe, others are not. Certain conditions and behaviors can make a safe area an unsafe one. The following suggestions will help you keep your baby safe.

- Place your baby on his back. Do not put your baby on his tummy or side.

- Remove all soft, fluffy, or loose bedding and toys from your baby's sleep area.

- Use only a lightweight cover or blanket. Do not use comforters, duvets, quilts, or pillows.

- Dress your baby in a single layer of clothing or a sleep sack. Do not let your baby get too hot.

- Place your baby on a firm mattress or other firm surface. Do not place your baby on a soft mattress, waterbed, sofa, or chair.

- Do not place your baby alone in an adult bed.

- Do not place your baby in an adult bed with older children.

- Parents who smoke should not sleep with their baby.

- Parents should not sleep with their baby if they have used alcohol or drugs.

- Parents should not sleep with their baby if they are overly tired.

- Parents who are very overweight should not sleep with their baby.

If you have questions about sleeping with your baby, talk with your baby's health care provider.

When will my baby sleep through the night?

After your baby is breastfeeding well and gaining weight, you can begin to let him set his own feeding schedule. This may happen at about 4–6 weeks after birth. Remember that every baby is different. Some babies will breastfeed every 2–3 hours, day and night, for many weeks. Others will breastfeed every 1–2 hours when awake and sleep for longer periods of time. By 6–12 weeks of age, many babies will sleep from midnight until 4 or 5 o'clock in the morning. You simply need to change your idea of night!

How can I stop my baby from crying?

Babies cry for lots of reasons, and some cry more than others. Sometimes it is easy to know the cause of the crying, but more often no cause is found. Many babies have a fussy period in the late afternoon or early evening. Some babies will stop crying if they are held, cuddled, rocked, or bathed. It takes time for you to know what works with your baby.

The best way to stop the crying is to check each of the likely causes. Your baby may be hungry, tired, cold, hot, bored, or sick. If he is hungry, feed him. If he is tired, place him in his crib. If he is fussy, try to hold, walk, or rock him. If he has a wet or dirty diaper, change it. If he is too hot, take his clothes off. If he is too cold, put some clothes on him. If he is sick, take his temperature. If he has a fever, take him to his health care provider or call the WIC clinic (see "What is WIC," p. 95).

If you find that you are unable to cope with your baby's crying, give him to someone else to care for and take a break. If this is not possible, put him safely in his crib and turn on some music or take a bath or do whatever helps you relax.

Can I give my baby a pacifier?

The more often you breastfeed, the sooner you and your baby will learn this important skill. If you use a pacifier in the early weeks, your baby may breastfeed less often, and may not learn to breastfed well. Some studies suggest that pacifiers may reduce the risk of sudden infant death syndrome (SIDS). But it is best to wait until your baby is breastfeeding well (about 4–6 weeks after birth) before offering a pacifier. Many breastfed babies prefer to suck on thumbs, fingers, or fists!

Do I need to give my baby vitamins?

Your baby needs a single dose of vitamin K and a daily dose of vitamin D. Vitamin K is given soon after birth, by your baby's doctor. Sunlight is the main source of vitamin D. Because the amount of sunlight your baby receives is hard to measure and because too much sunlight can be harmful, many doctors recommend that babies be given a dose of 200 IU of vitamin D each day beginning by 2 months of age.

How long should my baby breastfeed?

Some mothers breastfeed for a few weeks, some for a few months, and others for a few years. Any amount of breastfeeding is good for you and your baby. How long you breastfeed depends on your needs and the needs of your child.

 Breastmilk is the only food your baby needs for about the first 6 months.

Some babies start to lose interest in breastfeeding between 6 and 12 months when solid foods are offered. Replacing breastmilk with other foods is called weaning. More important than when you wean is that you wean slowly. Some babies wean completely between 12 and 24 months. Others continue to breast-feed on and off for 3, 4, or more years—the breast is a wonderful place to eat, sleep, and cuddle!

Hints for weaning slowly
- Replace one breastfeeding at a time with solids or liquids, depending on your baby's age and ability. You might want to ask another family member— perhaps your baby's brother, sister, or father—to offer the substitute.

- Replace one daily breastfeeding every 3–5 days until weaning is complete.

- Increase cuddling time. Your baby can still find comfort and safety in your arms.

- Keep an active toddler busy with games, outdoor play, and story-telling.

- Expect some milk production for many days or even many weeks after weaning is complete.

Sometimes something happens (accident or illness) and a mother needs to wean quickly.

Hints for weaning quickly
- Hand express or pump a small amount of milk to relieve fullness and prevent swelling. Remove only enough milk to relieve fullness. The more milk you remove, the more milk you will make.

- Put cold packs on the breasts to relieve pain and reduce swelling.

- Wear a snug bra for comfort and support.

- Take acetaminophen (Tylenol) or ibuprofen (Advil) for pain.

When should I give my baby solid foods?

Birth to 6 months
Breastmilk is the only food your baby needs for about the first 6 months of life. If you start solid foods too soon, you can cause constipation, diarrhea, gas, spitting-up, or allergy.

6 months to 1 year
When your baby is about 6 months old, you can begin to offer solid foods. You will know your baby is ready for solid foods if he can sit up, turn his head, put food in his mouth, and swallow. Even though solid foods provide vitamins and nutrients, breastmilk should be a key part of your baby's diet for at least 1 year.

If you stop breastfeeding before your baby is 1 year old, ask your baby's health care provider to recommend an iron-rich formula. Your baby should be 1 year old before you give him cow's milk.

What are growth spurts?

There may be times when your baby grows faster than usual. This is called a growth spurt. A sudden increase in the number of breastfeedings may signal a growth spurt. Growth spurts often occur around 3 weeks, 6 weeks, 3 months, and 6 months. But growth spurts can occur at any time. Because your baby wants to eat all the time, your family and friends may suggest that "you are not making enough milk," that "you need to give your baby solid foods or formula," or that "it is time to stop breastfeeding." Be patient. After 2–3 days, your milk supply will increase and your baby will ask to breastfeed less often.

What are nursing strikes?

A nursing strike is a sudden refusal to breastfeed. Sometimes the strike has a clear cause such as teething, fever, ear infection, stuffy nose (cold), constipation, or diarrhea. Deodorant, perfume, or powder placed on a mother's skin can also cause a strike. Sometimes no cause is found. You will need to hand express or pump your breasts until the strike ends. In the meantime, give your baby your expressed milk using a teaspoon, eye dropper, hollow-handled medicine spoon, or cup. Watch your baby for early signs of hunger and offer the breast at those times. Breastfeed in a quiet place. Give your baby your full attention. Nursing strikes seldom lead to weaning.

Breastfeeding Special Babies

Can I breastfeed if I have more than one baby?

Many mothers produce enough milk to meet the needs of two (or more) babies. The more milk your babies take from your breasts, the more milk you will make.

At first you may find it easier to feed one baby at a time. But after you and your babies have learned to breastfeed well, you can save time by feeding two babies at once. Some babies will breastfeed on one breast at a feeding, while others will breastfeed on both breasts. Just remember that each baby needs to breastfeed at least eight times in each 24 hours.

Two or more babies take more time no matter how you choose to feed them. So don't forget to take care of yourself as well as your babies. Eat a variety of healthy foods, drink enough fluid to satisfy your thirst, and accept all offers of help from family and friends.

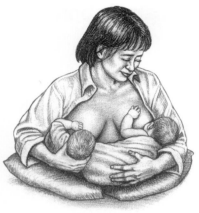

**COMBINATION CRADLE-
FOOTBALL/LAYERED/PARALLEL HOLD**

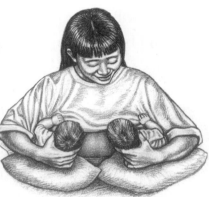

DOUBLE-FOOTBALL/DOUBLE-CLUTCH HOLD

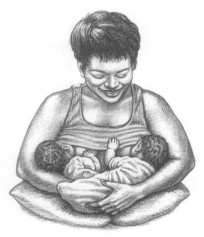

CRISS-CROSS/DOUBLE-CRADLE HOLD

Can I breastfeed if my baby is born early?

The birth of a tiny baby born weeks or months early can be scary. You may have many questions.

- Why did this happen?
- Was it something I did?
- How will he eat if he is too little to suck?
- Can I breastfeed?

Babies born early can be breastfed, even those needing special care. Breastfeeding gives parents a chance to share in the care of their baby and to do something that no one else can do. The milk of mothers who give birth early contains just the right amount of nutrients to meet the needs of even the earliest babies.

Let the hospital staff know that you plan to breastfeed. If your baby is too small or too sick to breastfeed, he can still be fed your milk. The hospital staff can show you how to express and store your milk.

As soon as your baby is well enough to be held for a period of time each day, ask his nurse if you can put him underneath your clothing and cuddle him skin-to-skin against your chest (kangaroo care).

Your baby's health care provider will let you know when your baby is ready to breastfeed.

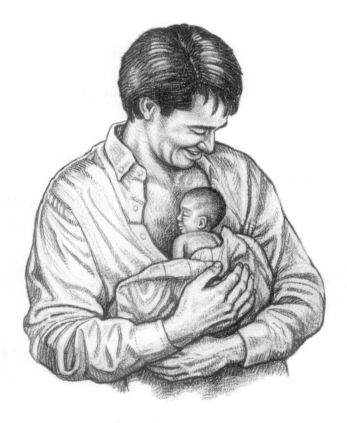

You can care for your baby by holding him skin-to-skin.

Can I breastfeed if I have a cesarean birth?

Mothers who have had a cesarean birth (C-section) can still breastfeed. If the mother or baby needs special care, the start of breastfeeding may be delayed. If you have had a cesarean birth, you may find the following suggestions helpful.

- Choose a comfortable position. Use extra pillows to protect the incision (cut) and provide support. The side-lying or football positions are best.

- Keep your baby in the room with you to save time and energy.

- Get plenty of rest. Nap when your baby naps.

- Limit your activity. Try not to do any heavy lifting, household chores, or brisk exercise for 4–6 weeks.

- Pain medicine may be necessary for several days. Your doctor will recommend medicine that is safe for you and your baby.

Taking Care of Yourself

What should I do if my breasts are swollen and hard?

During the first week after your baby is born, your milk supply will steadily increase and your breasts may feel full and heavy. Frequent breastfeeding will relieve the fullness, but if you delay or miss feedings your breasts can get swollen, hard, and painful.

Hints for relieving swollen breasts

- Hand express or pump a small amount of milk or colostrum. This will soften the breast and make it easier for your baby to latch on.

- Use cold packs between feedings to reduce the swelling. You can use bags of frozen peas wrapped in a cool, wet washcloth.

- Increase the flow of milk by gently squeezing the breast when your baby pauses from feeding.

- Breastfeed every 1–3 hours during the day and every 2–3 hours at night.

- Wear a bra for comfort and support, but make sure the bra fits well and is not too tight.

After several weeks, your milk supply will change to meet your baby's needs, and your breasts may seem smaller and less full. Do not worry, you are not losing your milk!

What should I do if my nipples are sore?

Your nipples may be tender during the first week when you and your baby are learning to breastfeed. Many mothers feel a tug or pull when their baby latches on to the breast. This is normal. Breastfeeding should not be painful if your baby is positioned well. If you feel pain for more than a few seconds, your baby may not have a good latch. Break the suction, remove your baby from the breast, and try again.

Hints for relieving sore nipples

- Begin each feeding on the breast that is least sore. If both breasts are sore, put a warm, wet washcloth on both breasts and use gentle massage to start the flow of milk.

- If your breasts are full and hard, express a small amount of milk or colostrum to soften the breast.

- Position your baby correctly on the breast. Remember, his chin should touch the breast and his mouth should be opened wide.

- Hold your baby close to prevent pulling on the nipples. Remember to break the suction before you take your baby off the breast.

- If necessary, breastfeed more often (every 1–2 hours) and for shorter periods of time (10–15 minutes or until the breast is soft).

- You don't need to wash your nipples before each breastfeeding. Even clear water, used often, will dry the skin.

- After each breastfeeding, put a small amount of breastmilk on the areola and nipple of each breast. To keep the skin moist you might want to use modified lanolin instead. A little bit goes a long way!

- If your nipples are painful, cracked, or bleeding, call your health care provider.

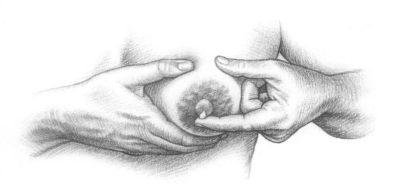

You can put a small amount of breastmilk on the nipple and areola after each feeding to ease soreness.

How can I keep my breasts from leaking?

Leaking sometimes occurs when you think about your baby, hear him or another baby cry, delay a feeding, or have sex.

Hints to control leaking

- You can stop the flow of milk by pressing the heels of your hands against your nipples or folding your arms across your chest.

- Use breast pads to protect your clothes. Change pads frequently, and do not use pads with plastic liners that trap wetness.

- To hide wetness, choose clothing with light colors and small prints.

Do I need to change what I eat?

You can eat all the foods you ate before! Eat a variety of foods—vegetables, fruits, bread, cereal, rice, pasta, meat, poultry, fish, beans, eggs, yogurt, milk, and cheese. Drink enough fluid so that you are not thirsty. Water, skim or low-fat milk, and unsweetened fruit juice are good choices. You will know that you are drinking enough fluid if your urine is clear or pale yellow in color.

Some mothers find that certain foods make their baby fussy. If this happens, simply stay away from that food.

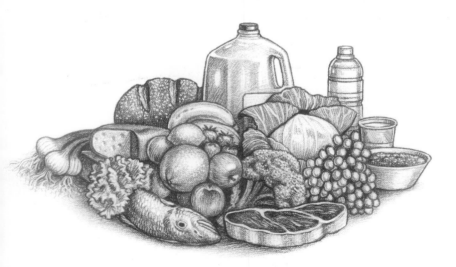

Keep yourself healthy by eating a variety of foods.

Can I drink alcohol?

 Alcohol (beer, wine, liquor) passes easily into breast-milk, and even small amounts can affect your ability to care for your baby. If you choose to drink alcohol, have no more than one or two drinks a week and wait at least 2 hours after you drink before breastfeeding.

Can I smoke or chew tobacco?

Smoke and nicotine can harm you and your baby. If
you smoke or chew tobacco and cannot stop, you can
still breastfeed. But do not smoke in the house or car
or near your baby.

Can I breastfeed if I take illegal ("street") drugs?

 Drugs that are sold on the street (crack, heroin, and marijuana) can harm you and your baby. Street drugs pass into your milk and to your baby. They can make it hard for your baby to eat, sleep, breathe, and grow. Mothers who take street drugs should not breastfeed.

Can I breastfeed and still lose weight?

Yes. Mothers who breastfeed often lose weight more easily than mothers who don't. This happens because some of the calories needed to make breastmilk come from the fat stored during pregnancy. The rest of the calories come from the foods you eat. Remember to eat a variety of healthy foods each day (vegetables, fruits, breads, cereals, meat, fish, poultry, eggs, milk, and cheese) and to exercise regularly.

To lose added pounds…

- drink nonfat or low-fat milk, water, or unsweetened fruit juice.

- limit cakes, cookies, pies, candy, and ice cream.

- snack on fresh fruits and raw vegetables.

- bake or broil meat and fish.

- exercise each day (walking, biking, running).

What if I get sick and need medicine?

Unless you have a serious illness like HIV/AIDS, the best protection for your baby is your breastmilk, so keep breastfeeding. Check with your doctor before you take any medicine, including medicine you buy over the counter (without a prescription). Make sure your doctor knows that you are breastfeeding so he or she can recommend medicine that is safe for you and your baby.

Take care of yourself and your baby. Keep your baby in the room with you and nap when he naps. Ask your family and friends to help with household chores. If you have to stay in the hospital, let the hospital staff know that you are breastfeeding and ask if your baby can stay with you. If you need to be away from your baby, you can pump your breasts to relieve fullness and to keep your milk supply. The hospital or WIC clinic may have a breast pump that you can use. (See "What is WIC," p. 95.) Most babies will breastfeed again when given the chance. If your baby refuses to breastfeed, ask your health care provider for help.

What about sex?

You may have little interest in sex at first. A new baby takes time and energy. Many women worry that sex will be painful or that they will get pregnant again. Let your partner know how you feel.

Before you have sex, talk with your doctor about birth control and choose a method that fits your lifestyle.

When you have sex, milk can leak from your breasts. It will help if you breastfeed your baby before you make love. This will give you more time for sex or sleep, whichever comes first!

When you breastfeed, your vagina (birth canal) may be dry, and sex can be uncomfortable. A lubricant like K-Y Jelly can be helpful. Put a small amount around the opening of the vagina before having sex.

Can I take birth control pills while I am breastfeeding?

Most women want to plan their pregnancies. If you wait at least a year before you get pregnant again, your body will have a chance to heal.

Birth control pills that contain estrogen can decrease your milk supply, but birth control pills that contain only progesterone are thought to be safe. Some mothers notice a decrease in their milk supply even when taking progesterone-only pills. So it is best to wait until you have a good supply of milk (at least 6 weeks after your baby is born) before taking pills that contain progesterone. If your milk supply decreases, talk with your doctor about another type of birth control. There are many choices, including natural family planning, diaphragm, sponge, vaginal ring, intrauterine device (IUD), condom, and spermicidal cream, foam, or jelly.

Can I get pregnant if I am breastfeeding?

Yes! If you breastfeed fully and never or almost never give your baby formula, water, or other foods, you are less likely to get pregnant. But if you give your baby formula, water, or other foods, or use a pacifier often, you are more likely to get pregnant. If you do not want to have another baby soon, talk with your doctor about birth control.

If I get pregnant, can I still breastfeed?

Yes! Many mothers continue to breastfeed an older baby while pregnant, and some older babies continue to breastfeed after the new baby is born. This is called "tandem nursing." In order to meet the nutritional needs of two babies as well as your own needs, eat a variety of healthy foods, drink to satisfy your thirst, and nap when the babies nap.

Returning to Work or School

Can I breastfeed after I go back to work or school?

Many mothers continue to breastfeed after they return to work or school. It takes a little extra planning, but the benefits are worth it!

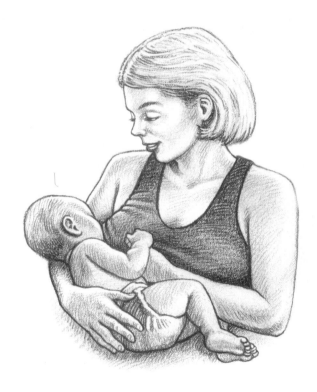

Continuing to breastfeed after you go back to school is easy. You just need to plan ahead.

- Breastfeeding keeps you and your baby close even when you are apart.
- Breastfed babies are healthier, even those in child care.
- Parents who breastfeed miss less work and lose less income.
- Breastfeeding saves time with no formula to mix, measure, or warm.
- Breastfeeding makes parents' lives simpler, especially for parents going back to work or school.

Learn how to express and collect your milk. If you plan to have your milk fed to your baby while you are apart, you will need to learn how to express and collect your milk. Practice early and often so that you learn this important skill before you return to work or school.

Decide who will take care of your baby. Choose a babysitter who...

- provides a safe, clean place for your baby.
- has taken care of breastfed babies before.
- understands and supports breastfeeding.
- is near your work or school if you wish to breast-feed during the day.

Introduce a bottle or cup. If you are going to be away from your baby during feeding times, you need to know that he will accept food from something other than the breast and from someone other than you. About 2 weeks before you return to work, offer

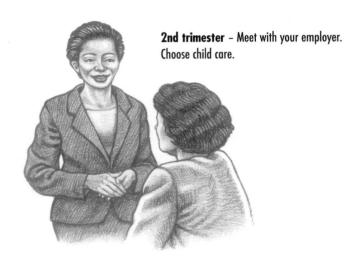

2nd trimester – Meet with your employer. Choose child care.

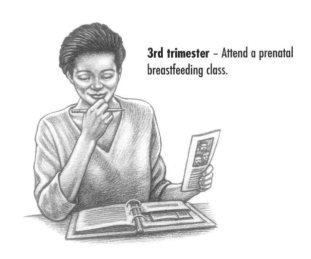

3rd trimester – Attend a prenatal breastfeeding class.

your baby your milk in a bottle or cup. (Babies can learn to cup feed at any age.) If you use a bottle, try different kinds of nipples until you find one that your baby will take. You may find it easier if someone other than you offers your expressed milk.

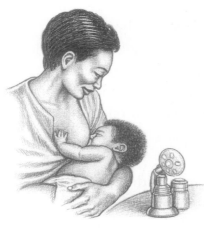

Birth - Breastfeed as soon as possible.

Week 1 - Breastfeed at least 8 times in each 24 hours.

Week 2 - Learn to express and collect your milk; freeze milk for later use.

Week 4 - Introduce a bottle or cup.

Weeks 6–12 - Delay your return to work for 12 weeks if possible.

2 weeks before you return to work - Decide how much time you will need each work day to get yourself and your baby ready.

1 week before you return to work - Hold a dress rehearsal.

After you return to work - Make the most of your time together.

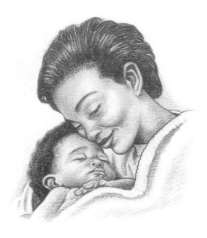

How do I express my milk?

You can express your milk by hand or with a pump. If you will need to express often or for many weeks or months, you can rent or buy an electric pump with a special kit that lets you pump both breasts at the same time.

At first, you may get only enough milk to cover the bottom of the collection container. Don't worry! It may take several days before you see an increase in the amount of milk expressed. Try to relax and think about your baby.

Hints for expressing your milk with a pump
You can express milk from one breast while your baby breastfeeds from the other breast, or you can express milk between feedings. When your baby breastfeeds, a let-down reflex occurs. Mothers who pump while breastfeeding often get more milk. If your baby is unable to keep up with the added flow of milk, he will pull away from the breast for several seconds until the flow slows down. You may want to keep a cloth handy to soak up the milk!

- Before you start, wash your hands with soap and water and rinse well.

- Follow the directions that come with your pump.

- Express for 5–10 minutes or until the flow of milk slows down. Rest for 3–5 minutes, and then repeat once or twice.

- Express each breast until the flow of milk slows down and the breast softens.

- Wash the pump after each use in hot, soapy water and rinse well.

- At work or school, rinse the pump in hot water. Wash in hot, soapy water when you get home.

Hints for expressing your milk by hand
- Press your breast against your chest, and then gently squeeze your breast between your thumb and fingers.

- Move your thumb and fingers around the breast until all parts of the breast are soft and the flow of milk slows down.

Hints to make expression easier
- Choose a quiet, comfortable place.

- Put warm, wet washcloths on your breasts.

- Massage your breasts in a circular motion.
- Relax and think about your baby.
- Listen to a relaxation tape or music tape.
- Look at a picture of your baby.
- Eat a healthy snack.

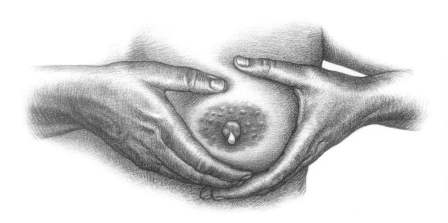

Hand expression is inexpensive and easy.

You can store your milk in any container made for food. Use something that is not likely to break, tear, or tip over in the refrigerator or freezer. There are even plastic storage bags made just for breastmilk. Place the container of milk in a refrigerator or freezer, or store it in a thermos or cooler.

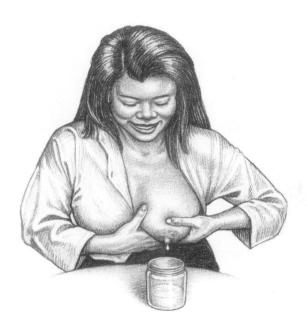

You can express your milk into any container
that has a wide opening and is made for food.

How do I choose a breast pump?

Wait until after your baby is born to buy or rent a breast pump. You may find that plans made during pregnancy change. Here are some things to consider when choosing a breast pump...

- Why do you need a breast pump?
- How often do you plan to pump?
- Is the pump comfortable?
- Is the pump easy to use?
- Is the pump easy to clean?
- How much does the pump cost?

There are different types of pumps: manual (hand) pumps, battery-operated pumps, semi-automatic electric pumps, and automatic (self-cycling) electric pumps. Whether you plan to pump two or three times a day or two or three times a week, you should choose a pump that is comfortable and easy to use. The pump should provide gentle compression of the breast and removal of milk with the least amount of vacuum. Milk expression should be quick, easy, and painless! Important features include adjustable vacuum, back-flow protection, and double-pumping capability. The more expensive pumps are available for sale or rent.

How long can I store my milk?

Handle your breastmilk the same way you care for other foods. Store your milk in a cool place, refrigerate it as soon as possible, and freeze it for later use. If you are storing milk for a healthy, full-term baby, follow these simple suggestions.

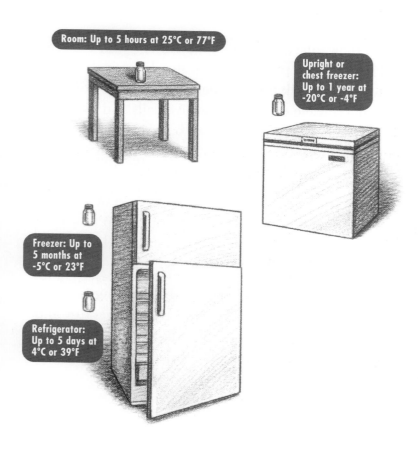

Room: Up to 5 hours at 25°C or 77°F

Upright or chest freezer: Up to 1 year at -20°C or -4°F

Freezer: Up to 5 months at -5°C or 23°F

Refrigerator: Up to 5 days at 4°C or 39°F

- Store your milk in any container made for food. Label the container with your name, your baby's name, the date, and the time. Place a single serving in each container.

- Recommended storage times vary. To be safe, store your milk in a cool room for up to 5 hours, in the refrigerator for up to 5 days, in the freezer section of a refrigerator/freezer for up to 5 months, or in an upright or chest freezer for up to 1 year. If you forget storage times, simply count the number of fingers on one hand as a reminder—five!

- To thaw, place the unopened container in the refrigerator or in a pan of warm water. Do not thaw or warm any milk for your baby in a microwave oven. A microwave oven destroys live cells and heats the milk unevenly. Hot milk can burn your baby.

- Milk that has been thawed in the refrigerator should be used within 24 hours. Milk that has been thawed in a pan of warm water should be used right away or stored in the refrigerator for up to 4 hours. Any milk left in the feeding container (e.g., bottle or cup) should be thrown away.

- Breastmilk is easy to prepare. No heating is needed. Simply remove the milk from the refrigerator and serve. If your baby prefers milk at room temperature, place the unopened container in a pan of warm water for several minutes.

Getting Help

Where can I find help with breastfeeding?

There are many health professionals to whom you can turn for help including WIC nutritionists, International Board Certified Lactation Consultants, La Leche League Leaders, and breastfeeding peer counselors. Family and friends who have breastfed can also be a source of much-needed encouragement and support. If you or your baby has a medical problem, contact your doctor or your baby's doctor right away.

What is WIC?

WIC (the Special Supplemental Nutrition Program for Women, Infants and Children) is a special government nutrition program that provides healthy foods and nutrition counseling to low-income women who are pregnant, have recently given birth, or are breastfeeding, and to children up to age 5 years. Nearly 50 percent of babies born in the United States participate in WIC. WIC nutritionists, nurses, and peer counselors serve between 7 and 8 million women and children each month.

How do I qualify for WIC?

Your income must be below a certain level, you must live in an area that has a WIC clinic, and you must be "at nutritional risk." A health professional will determine whether a woman or child is at nutritional risk.

If your income allows you to participate in the Food Stamp, Medicaid, or Temporary Assistance to Needy Families (TANF) programs, you would meet the income requirement for WIC, but you must also meet the residency requirement and be at nutritional risk to qualify for WIC.

What foods does WIC provide?

WIC foods include fruit and vegetable juices, cereal, eggs, milk, cheese, peanut butter, dried beans, infant formula, and infant cereal. Most WIC clinics give you a check or voucher so that you can buy the foods at a nearby grocery store. Some WIC clinics ask you to pick up the foods at a warehouse. Other clinics deliver the foods to your home.

How does WIC help breastfeeding mothers?

- Women who breastfeed can participate in WIC until their babies are 1 year of age. Women who formula-feed can participate only until their babies are 6 months of age.

- Women who breastfeed receive more foods for themselves and their families.

- Knowing that breastfeeding is the best choice for babies, WIC staff encourage and support breast-feeding.

- Some WIC clinics employ lactation consultants and peer counselors who provide breastfeeding support during and after your pregnancy.

- Some WIC clinics provide breast pumps so that mothers can continue to breastfeed after returning to work or school.

To find a WIC clinic in your area, check with your local health department or contact…

USDA Food and Nutrition Service
Public Affairs Staff
Tel: (703) 305-2286
Website: fns.usda.gov/wic

What is an International Board Certified Lactation Consultant?

An International Board Certified Lactation Consultant (IBCLC) is a health care provider with special knowledge and skills in breastfeeding management. To become an IBCLC, an individual must pass a test given by the International Board of Lactation Consultant Examiners.

IBCLCs work in hospitals, WIC clinics, and doctors' offices, and in private practice. An IBCLC can give you confidence in your ability to breastfeed and help you manage any problems that may occur.

To find an International Board Certified Lactation Consultant (IBCLC) in your area, contact...

International Lactation Consultant Association
1500 Sunday Drive, Suite 102
Raleigh, NC 27607
Tel: (919) 787-5181
Fax: (919) 787-4916
E-mail: ilca@erols.com
Website: ilca.org

What is a La Leche League Leader?

A La Leche League Leader is an experienced mother who has breastfed her own children for at least one year and who has been trained to answer your breast-feeding questions. To become a La Leche League Leader, an individual must be accredited by La Leche League International, an organization with the sole purpose of helping mothers breastfeed. La Leche League Leaders are representatives of La Leche League International and serve as volunteers.

To find a La Leche League Leader in your area, contact...

La Leche League International
1400 North Meacham Road
Schaumburg, IL 60168-4079
Tel: (800) 525-3243
Fax: (847) 519-0035
E-mail: LLLHQ@llli.org
Website: lalecheleague.org

What is a breastfeeding peer counselor?

A breastfeeding peer counselor is a mother who has breastfed her own children and helps mothers in her community breastfeed. To become a breastfeeding peer counselor, an individual must complete a breast-feeding peer counselor training program. Breastfeed-ing peer counselors may work as volunteers or be paid by an agency.

To find a breastfeeding peer counselor in your area, contact your local hospital, health department, or WIC clinic.

What does that word mean?

Alveoli: Alveoli are groups of cells inside the breast that make milk.

Antibodies: Antibodies are special proteins that protect you and your baby from infection.

Areola: The areola is the darker part of the breast around the nipple.

Colostrum: Colostrum is the first milk your breasts make.

Let-down reflex: The release of milk from the breast is called the let-down reflex.

Milk duct: Milk ducts are small tubes that carry milk from the milk-producing cells (alveoli) to the openings in the nipple.

Montgomery's gland: Montgomery's glands are small, pimple-like bumps in the darker part of the breast (areola) around the nipple.

About the Author

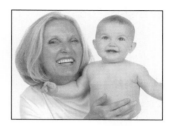

Amy Spangler, MN, RN, IBCLC, is a wife, mother, nurse, lactation consultant, educator, and author. She earned her bachelor's degree in nursing from the Ohio State University and her master's degree in maternal and infant health from the University of Florida. Amy is a registered nurse, an International Board Certified Lactation Consultant, a former president of the International Lactation Consultant Association, and a former chair of the United States Breastfeeding Committee. Amy has worked with mothers, babies, and families for over 30 years. She and her husband live in Atlanta, Georgia, and have two sons.

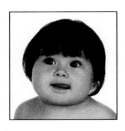

**For more information about our products,
please contact:**
Amy's Babies
P.O. Box 501046
Atlanta, GA 31150-1046
Tel: (770) 913-9332
Fax: (770) 913-0822
E-mail: amyspangler@amysbabies.com
Website: amysbabies.com